THE CARNIVORE DIET

THE BEST KEPT SECRETS OF HOW TO FEEL GREAT, TAKE CONTROL OF YOUR WEIGHT AND UNLEASH YOUR INNER CARNIVORE

ROBERT F. DURANT

ZENITH PUBLISHING

ZENITH PUBLISHING

First published in this edition 2019

ISBN-13: 9781710305029

Contents

THE

CARNIVORE

DIET

THE BEST KEPT SECRETS OF HOW TO FEEL GREAT, TAKE CONTROL OF YOUR WEIGHT AND UNLEASH YOUR INNER CARNIVORE

WHAT IS THE CARNIVORE DIET?

To be a carnivore is to eat meat: That is all it means, it's a concept that to many of us will feel strange and counter intuitive, and as such when it comes to dieting and weight loss, eating only animal products that are high in healthy fats and low in carbohydrates definitely comes with questions. The carnivore diet is based on the nutrition of our prehistoric ancestors; a time period when humanity was healthy, natural, and entirely unexposed to chemical additives.

Around 12,000 years ago the human race transitioned from its hunter-gatherer lifestyle into a modern agricultural society in which the diet changed from one focused on animal-based fats and protein to a diet that consisted almost exclusively of carbohydrates. We don't know why our ancestors made the decision to change to an agricultural society, but we do know that large communities and cities would not be able to develop without this change. Prior to this transition, the typical hunter-gatherer required approximately 10 square miles to hunt effectively, whereas a pre-historic farmer needed only a tenth of a square mile to feed themselves. Since then, we have been adapting the environment and the food we eat to cater to our needs with less effort and fewer resources, the result has been a plant-based diet that is abundant with simple carbohydrates and chemical pesticides. Our bodies and instincts were adapted for the stone age, and as such this was the last time that we ate an entirely healthy diet without having to think about it.

During the Paleolithic era, a period ranging from 2.6 million years ago to 12,000 years ago, the agricultural revolution had not yet occurred, and humankind had to forage for what they could find, this meant fresh, natural ingredients, with meat being a primary source of nutrition. In modern times, scientists have come to realize that our diets had diverged far from the healthy sources of nutrition that our diet used to contain. While we'll discuss later the issues surrounding added sugars, processed grains and carbohydrates, the main idea behind the carnivore diet is that humankind used to be healthier, stronger, and that their diets were a significant factor that enabled them to endure the harsh conditions of prehistoric life- in short it was a diet their bodies were evolved for and allowed them to perform at their physical peak. While you probably are not hunting down a mastodon out in the plains, there are men who still output the same, if not more, physical activity every day than our Paleolithic counterparts, so why wouldn't the same diet work to sustain a healthier lifestyle in the modern world?

Scientists have discovered that our bodies are equipped with a vestigial catabolic mechanism that allows us to burn different types of fuel to maximize our nutrition and muscle growth. Catabolic is the adjective that describes any process that breaks down an initial material to harvest energy from it. When we choose to fuel our bodies with foods that are high in healthy fats (like meat), but low in carbohydrates, we trigger this mechanism to start a chain of processes that result in weight loss and energy delivery that will revolutionize the way your body performs. While we'll dive into the scientific details on carbohydrate-free catabolism later in this book, you should be getting the sense by now that the carnivore diet is a lifestyle that seeks to return the human body to its natural state from a dietary perspective.

You may be familiar with other nutrition plans based on prehistoric diets, particularly the paleo diet, which allows for the consumption of other foods that were available to prehistoric humans such as nuts, fruits and vegetables. The carnivore diet, which only allows the consumption of animal based foods, differs from these diets for two main reasons: Firstly, many of the natural foods available to our ancestors are almost unrecognizable to us today as a result of modern agriculture, typically the sweetest form of fruit available to prehistoric man would be as sweet as a modern carrot and so if we were to include these in the regime, we would not able to reflect a prehistoric diet accurately, furthermore the inclusion of modern plant based foods encourages the consumption of too many sources of carbohydrate rich foods. Secondly, the Paleolithic diet is improved by the exclusion of plant-based foods, for reasons we will go into later in this book the consumption of these foods can have negative health effects, and a 100%

animal-based diet will offer greater nutrition overall.

It is important to note that carbohydrates are not inherently bad for us, even though the majority of publicly accepted nutritional science has been found to be incorrect, especially with respect to how much of our diet should incorporate carbohydrates. Models such as the carbohydrate-dominated food pyramid, which introduced in 1992, have focused on people shifting their food choices from red meats and healthy fats to carbohydrate laden diets. Shortly before the introduction of the food-pyramid, in 1990, the obesity rate in the USA was at 11.1%, in 2017 the obesity rate was found to be 30.6%, that is, that 3 in 10 Americans are obese. The war on fat of the 1980s, and the introduction of government advice promoting a high carbohydrate diet have done nothing but increase the amount of people that do not have control of their weight. The science behind a carbohydrate-based diet has been shown to be ineffective. That is not to say that carbohydrates cannot be present in a healthy diet, especially when they occur in naturally low amounts, such as the low levels of carbohydrates found in meat.

Your body's preferred sources of fuel are glucose sugars, but even though your body gives preference to this source of energy, it is not the most efficient way for the human body to absorb, convert, and use nutritional energy. Healthy fats provide almost three times the amount of energy as carbohydrates, and when we eat too many, they aren't stored as the by-product glycogen in our fat cells. Eating only healthy fats doesn't just lower your cholesterol, regulate your blood pressure, and maintain a stable blood sugar. When you eat only fats, your body will enter into a ketogenic state in which your body will undergo a process called ketosis, which boosts your energy, stimulates cognitive function, and allows your muscles to grow stronger faster. Although it might sound too good to be true, you are entirely capable of healthily shifting your body's fuel source and still consuming all the micronutrients that your body requires by eating only animal sourced products.

A low carbohydrate carnivore diet is the eating plan that will help you take control of your weight, nutrition and fitness. Ultimately this plan is more than just a weight-loss diet, and while it will help you to get in shape and lose those pounds you should approach this as a new lifestyle, and while it may appear restrictive at first, after experiencing the benefits, you'll never want to go back.

How the human diet changed for the worst

Our diets as a species have undergone drastic changes in the past few centuries, and it's no surprise that as our lives have become easier and more focused on convenience that we have forgotten that nutrition has always been one of the most important factors in our wellbeing. During the twentieth century, America had developed a booming fast food industry that appealed to our appetites and provided us with fast, convenient and delicious food.

As demand for food skyrocketed, it became necessary to create larger supply chains for the food we eat, at the same time we were developing appetites for foods that did not grow locally, as a result we were demanding foods from thousands of miles away that couldn't withstand the journey. In order to combat the natural process of decay, the food industry began using preservatives that would allow our food to last longer on the shelves and come from further away. For example, In a process called hydrogenation, fats and oils can be heated up to a temperature that somewhat solidifies their molecular structure, allowing them to last longer on the shelves before going bad, but hydrogenated fats and oils are not the same as the healthy fats and oils that they started out to be. Instead of offering our bodies a fatty acid fuel source that produces high energy ketones, these hydrogenated fats and oils are what we would now call saturated fats. Saturated fats are no longer the healthy monounsaturated sources that they began as, and they have the added effect of increasing your harmful low-density lipoprotein cholesterol levels, while actively reducing your good high-density lipoprotein cholesterol.

The final benefit of a carnivore diet that relates to an unhealthy development in agricultural farming is the lack of pesticides you will ingest when you are only eating animal sourced products. Plants are much more susceptible to natural predators like insects, and when maximizing the profit of every crop is a farmer's priority, it's no surprise that excessive amounts of pesticides are used. Our plants are often covered in chemicals that are designed to prevent them from being eaten by insects, but this often means using a spray that is poisonous. While most of these chemicals have passed heavy regulatory standards, it still doesn't mean that in the long term these chemicals are not having an effect on our bodies in the long term.

THE CARNIVORE DIET & THE BODY

In order to properly execute an effective carnivore diet, you will need to understand the processes that your body undergoes in order to enter into a ketogenic state.

Firstly, we will examine your metabolism and what happens when you switch from catabolizing carbs to catabolizing fats. Following this, we'll discuss the components of the Krebs cycle that make your body biologically primed for weight loss. Once you understand how your body needs to be fueled on a carnivore diet, you can maximize your gains, productivity, and weight loss based on only your fuel source. Theoretically, you will lose weight on the carnivore diet even without an exercise plan, because the science is designed to cut your body fat no matter what. But don't worry – we'll give you all the tips to make your carnivore eating work best for your lifestyle.

Defining your metabolism

Metabolic rate is a concept which is often poorly understood, and in many cases mistaken, at a huge detriment to your weight loss. Your metabolism is defined as the entirety of all of the chemical processes occurring within your body that you have to perform every day to stay alive. A fundamental misunderstanding of the concept of metabolism can create an incorrect mindset that can lead to fueling your body with the wrong composition of macronutrients. An incorrect balance of fuel that attempts to control your weight loss only tends to miss the point of a functioning metabolism.

When your body is operating normally, it catabolizes glucose first and foremost. Glucose is absorbed by the body through the digestive system and is broken down in our cells in order to release its energy. Within our cells are the mitochondria, also known as the powerhouse of the cell, these need glucose present inside the cells in order to break it down for energy.

The difficulty with this is that glucose molecules are too large to be absorbed into the cell without assistance, and such requires an additional hormone to help the glucose molecules pass through the cell membranes and into the cell, this hormone is insulin. One of insulin's main functions is to operate as a mechanism that fits into your cell walls to allow large glucose molecules to pass into the mitochondria. Insulin is secreted by the pancreas and acts principally to regulate the intake of sugar into our cells where it is then processed to release energy, and as a result your pancreas releases more insulin into your blood stream when the body recognizes that food is being digested.

Now, what does this have to do with your metabolism and your diet? Many Americans have one, both, or even more of the following conditions that are considered metabolic disorders: Type 2 and Type 1 diabetes, obesity, heart disease, and glucose galactose malabsorption disorder. The reasons most Americans *have* one of these disorders is because of the high amount of processed sugars, saturated fats, and hydrogenated oils in their diet. Most of these unhealthy elements started out healthy before being chemically altered to change their molecular structure. While this most often occurs in order to make foods last longer, it is also used in order to enhance the taste of nutritionally devoid meals.

On a carnivore diet, you are going to be eating mostly natural animal fats, which often contain no chemical additives or preservatives and have not been processed. It's important to note that a carnivore diet often doesn't include ingredients other than those that are animal sourced, such as meat, dairy, eggs and fat. The exception to this is a small amount of spice which is permitted and considered to have no nutritional implications on the diet as a whole but will make the lifestyle more enjoyable. In addition to this, salt is also an important addition to your diet as it is essential for good health.

When you fuel your body with only healthy fats, you are providing your body nearly three times the nutritional energy that you could with that same amount of carbohydrates. This means that your metabolism suddenly has an increased and more accessible supply of energy, without the side effects and fatigue that are associated with consuming too much glucose. From weight loss to cardiac function and digestive regularity, a carnivore diet effects every single aspect of your metabolism and is more than just a weight-loss regime, it's a lifestyle that's been tailored to optimize your metabolism to work better for longer.

Fat burning and the Krebs cycle

You already know that the breakdown of glucose takes place within the mitochondria of the cells, but there's another process that occurs within cellular respiration that's going to change the way you eat for the rest of your life. The Krebs cycle, also known as the citric acid cycle, is one of the oldest catabolic pathways in your body.

When you only fuel your body with healthy fats, your body will not have a ready supply of glucose in the bloodstream and so your cellular respiration has to run with triglyceride molecules instead of glucose, which you then turn into the fatty acids that will enter the Krebs cycle. Triglyceride is the scientific term for what we would usually call a fat molecule, but once they've been turned into fatty acid, triglycerides provide your body with almost three times the amount of energy when compared to a glucose molecule. Now, energy production is not the only reason that fat catabolism can be better than sugar; catabolizing fats also helps you to burb body fat without any effort.

Think back to what happens when you digest too much sugar – it gets stored as glycogen in your liver cells, muscle cells, and fat cells. However, healthy fats won't be stored in your body, both because they can't and because your body doesn't want to. When you eat too much fat, you produce an acidic bi-product during the Krebs cycle called a ketone body, a fuel for your brain and body that is not glucose-based.

On a glucose-free diet, your metabolism will go into glucose starvation mode, and your body will begin to seek out and burn those more difficult deep-tissue fatty sections that are so imbedded in our physique. On a low carb, high fat diet, you will almost always be able to achieve this fat burning ketogenic state. While this is difficult for some people because of the starches and sugars hidden in many healthy fruits and vegetables, individuals enjoying a carnivore diet barely have to think to ensure they don't consume any sugars. Since you will be eating only animal sourced foods like eggs, cheeses, and fatty meats, it's almost an afterthought to consider how much glucose you're consuming since your diet makes it almost non-existent.

Thinking about and maintaining ketogenic eating is one of the hardest parts of the keto diet, and it's one of the main reasons that most people don't make it through to the fat burning stage. You will be more likely to give up a carbohydrate diet if you're still consistently eating the sugary fruits and starchy vegetables that your body craves because it still wants its access to glucose. If you're still eating carbs, you can be sure you will also continue to experience carbohydrate withdrawal side effects. Eating a carnivorous diet in order to promote fat burning ketosis is easy, which makes for the most flexible and maintainable style of diets. In case you are not quite sold on why fruits and vegetables won't always be your best choice, let's examine the unhealthy plant toxins that might be damaging your health.

Why plants are not always best

For many animals, plants are their prey, and unlike other forms of prey they are unable to outrun their predators. However, plants have found an ingenious way of protecting themselves and that is by making themselves poisonous to their predators, and as a result they produce toxin proteins within their fibrous structures in order to protect themselves.

Almost every type of plant contains some sort of protein toxin. High concentrations of naturally occurring plant toxins can be found in almost all of our current produce. For example, leafy green vegetables, such as spinach and kale, often contain high levels of a poisonous chemical called oxalate. Oxalate is a chemical that plants use to store calcium. When you eat any one of these plants in any amount, you might think you are ingesting much more calcium than you are – because it's already being held onto by something else. Oxalates can cause damage all over your body, from interrupting your sleep cycles to causing phantom pain, carpal tunnel, and attention deficit disorder. Oxalates are easy to flush out of your system, but once they're already there, the damage is done, and it will take longer for your body to recover. Plants can also contain chemicals that interfere with human hormones, and there are more than a few reasons to support eliminating plants from your diet.

The benefits of a carnivore diet

A low carbohydrate diet fuels your body with high energy ketones that help you better rest, recover, and repair. For this reason, it's the perfect eating plan for anyone with a health issue that needs extra support. You already know that one of the first and most obvious benefits of a carnivore diet is intense and sustained healthy weight loss without physical effort. However, one of the other important benefits of a state of ketosis is increased energy to your muscles during workouts, clearer brain function due to a more powerful fuel source, as well as deeper sleep and more effective autophagy.

A low carbohydrate ketogenic diet triggers your body's mechanism of autophagy to more effectively clean and care for your tissues. Autophagy generally happens at night, and it's a gentle form of biological cell cannibalism. When we undergo what's called oxidative stress, a natural process that increases with aging, our cells become damaged and some no longer work. Your body uses other living cells to track down these broken vessels and catabolize their parts for use elsewhere in your body. Autophagy is the only thing that can reverse these aging-related malfunctions.

Everything about a carnivore diet promotes healthy and effective autophagy - including your sleep patterns. When you first start to eat a carnivore diet, you are going to experience some side effects based on something called a carbohydrate flu. This flu tends to operate like withdrawal symptoms when you no longer allow your body access to glucose – but like withdrawal, the symptoms end. Most people report sleeping badly during their flu period, but this only last a few days, and once full ketosis sets in, it's highly likely you will have never slept better.

When your body is burning ketones only, dieters find that they sleep longer hours, can stay asleep much better than they used to, and often engage in longer, deeper periods of restless eye movement, or REM, sleep. Our body's sleep patterns are controlled by our circadian rhythms, and they're about as ancient as our Krebs cycle pathway. Your circadian rhythm is

22

what responds to the rising of the sun in the morning to wake you up, and what put you to sleep as the night gets darker. However, your circadian rhythms also control a crucial release of energy into your bloodstream that occurs around four a.m. – a biological jumpstart that most of us didn't even know happened. Our circadian rhythms release a certain amount of insulin around four a.m. each morning to unlock stored glycogen and give us a significant boost in energy first thing in the morning. However, if your circadian rhythms are off, your body doesn't know when the appropriate time for this energy jolt is. As a result, you might not benefit, and a lack of morning energy isn't the only thing bad sleeping habits can affect. Once you enter into full ketosis, you will sleep deeper, and longer, but wake up earlier and more refreshed than you've been used to. Carnivore dieters with insomnia often chose to keep eating meat for the rest of their lives because it's the only time they've been able to achieve an effective sleep pattern.

The final benefit we're going to touch on associated with the carnivore diet relates back to your boosted metabolism but in relation to your testosterone levels and overall libido. Men who eat a more carbohydrate packed diet tend to feel not only sluggish in the gym, but sluggish everywhere else. When your body is not getting enough energy from a proper healthy food source, it's going to make compromises in order to maximize the use of whatever good nutrition you are actually getting. Most of the time for men older than twenty-five, a bad diet can have a huge effect on your libido and overall testosterone levels. A low carbohydrate diet that is high in healthy fats and stimulates ketosis will also stimulate your levels of testosterone and boost your libido. While elevating your testosterone levels is one of the best ways to boost your libido naturally, testosterone benefits your body in more ways than just reproductively.

Testosterone levels that are too low often cause depression, weakened bones that can degrade into osteoporosis, and the breakdown of lean muscle mass that contributes to muscular atrophy. Your testosterone levels are incredibly important, especially as you get older. Commonly referred to in the medical world as Low T, dangerously minimal testosterone levels will only get worse as you age and undergo more and more oxidative stress. Eating a consistent carnivore diet can vastly increase your testosterone levels anywhere from 13% to 29%. It can be a useful method in ensuring a lifetime of high testosterone and consistent libido when you choose to make an animal sourced, meat-based carnivore diet part of your long-term health solution.

Reversing and curing diseases with a low carbohydrate diet

If you think back to our discussion on metabolic disorders, you might start to see why eating a carnivore diet could be a great way to reverse certain medical disorders. The classic description of the Atkin's diet which was developed in the nineteen twenties is a low carbohydrate diet that is designed to combat seizures in epilepsy patients. The theory behind a low carbohydrate diet for epilepsy patients relies on the ability of fats to be broken down without stimulating seizures. When children at a young age diagnosed with epilepsy fasted intermittently or ate on a low carb diet (both eating patterns that trigger ketosis), scientists found that their seizures didn't occur when their bodies ran on ketone bodies but began to reoccur when proteins and carbohydrates were present in their diets.

For adults, the Atkin's diet was designed similarly to help adults manage epilepsy as well as high blood pressure, heart disease, and diabetes. Let's start with the carnivore diet and high blood pressure in relation to heart disease. When you eat too much unhealthy glucose, you raise your levels of bad low-density lipoprotein cholesterol and lower your levels of good high-density lipoprotein cholesterol. Cholesterol is a necessary fat-like steroid hormone that is designed to clear out the arteries around your heart. Good high-density lipoprotein cholesterol breaks down and removes plaque from difficult and clogged arteries so that your heart won't have to pump extra hard in order to properly circulate your blood. Atherosclerosis, or the tightening of your heart muscles as a result of high blood pressure, is one of the most common disorders effecting everyday Americans.

Eating a fatty diet high in animal sourced foods will allow you to control your cholesterol levels more accurately than if you were attempting to regulate them with only a regular diet and medication. Most patients eating on a low carbohydrate diet can take themselves off their blood pressure medication after approval from their doctor and months of clean, carnivorous eating.

Remember when we discussed autophagy? The reason those dead cells building up in your tissues become so harmful is that they cause inflammation in your tissues, and you would be surprised at the number of diseases caused by mere inflammation. Depression and anxiety are often linked to high levels of inflamed tissues, which are much less obvious symptoms of a tissue disorder. Arthritis or swelling of the joints due to autoimmune disorders as well as simple muscle soreness after a hard workout can all benefit immensely from eating a diet that cleans and clears out tough inflammation. But inflammation is not the only area that a carnivorous diet can improve. When you fuel your body with ketones, you should expect to experience a sharper mind with more focused concentration because of the neurological benefits of the carnivore diet.

The neurological effects of eating meat

Although depression and anxiety have proven to be amplified by inflammation, the neurological sources of each disorder can be occasionally unknown. However, autoimmune disorders that deal specifically with the neurons of the brain like multiple sclerosis, Alzheimer's, and Parkinson's disease have all shown scientifically correlated improvements in patients on extremely low carbohydrate diets. One of the most important benefits for busy individuals eating on a low carbohydrate diet is the incredible mental clarity that comes with fueling your brain with highly efficient ketones.

Many dieters that chose to switch to catabolizing fats report that they've never been as focused or as productive as they are when they're eating a carnivore diet. Your neurons are able to fire faster, work more efficiently, and repair themselves twice as efficiently as when your brain is functioning on ketones.

Low carbohydrate diets and type 2 diabetes

Type 2 diabetes is often caused by an unhealthy diet, obesity, or high blood sugar. The disease results in an inability to produce or regulate your insulin levels. You will recall that the pancreas releases insulin into the bloodstream when the body senses that we have consumed food. The more insulin that is present in your bloodstream, the more sugar your body will absorb during digestion. However, if your blood sugar is consistently high, you run the risk of over-working your pancreas and developing a dangerous inability to produce insulin. No insulin means a high concentration of glucose left in your bloodstream.

In the context of the carnivore diet, when you choose to fuel your body only with animal sourced fats and protein, there will be almost no glucose available to spike your blood sugar. Nutrients like healthy fats and proteins also tend to slow down your digestion, which allows your body to slowly and safely absorb your nutrients without spiking your blood sugar. It's worth mentioning that processed foods, and foods high in sugary additives, travel quickly through your digestive system, spiking your blood sugar and wreaking havoc on your digestion. This is simply another way that a meat-only diet can regulate your insulin levels, but it's worth it to note that the effects of ketosis can actually help reverse the effects of type 2 diabetes.

Who should not eat a meat-only diet?

The health benefits of the carnivore diet for regular individuals cannot be overstated, but there are specific medical conditions and biological predeterminations that make a meat-only diet dangerous. Although patients with type 2 diabetes can and should eat a low carbohydrate diet to manage their health, patients with the genetic form of the disease, type 1 diabetes, should never cut out carbohydrates. Type 1 diabetes differs from type 2 diabetes in that your body cannot produce insulin at all, and so you have to offer yourself intravenous injections to maintain stable blood sugar. Diabetics who are afflicted with type 1 tend to be more at risk of falling into a hypoglycemic coma, which occurs because of an insulin shock when your levels dip too low.

A diet that is high in healthy fats like a carnivore diet will already drastically reduce the amount of insulin in your bloodstream, and if you don't take the proper care to maintain your own blood sugar, your body won't be able to. Other patients who should avoid a carnivore diet are individuals with a history of eating disorders. The carnivore diet is designed to regulate your eating without limiting your nutrition, but any diet plan has the potential to trigger unhealthy habits. If you have a history of a heart condition as well, either a stroke, heart attack, or heart murmur, you should consult with your doctor before beginning a carnivore diet.

Managing your energy on the carnivore diet

One of the main reasons that individuals tend not to last on a carnivore diet is because they can't withstand the troughs in their energy levels. While most regular ketogenic dieters will experience more variation in energy levels than carnivorous dieters, you will still want to know the following tips and tricks to keep yourself energized. When you're eating carnivorously, you will be holding your body in a maintained state of ketosis.

One method that many carnivores like to use to combat their dips in energy is with something called bulletproof coffee. Bulletproof, or keto coffee, is made with full fat butter and natural whole coffee beans. Butter in your coffee or tea might sound a bit off-putting, but you will barely notice anything more than creamier texture than usual. Coffee that is packed with healthy fats first thing in the morning will help jumpstart your ketogenic mechanisms and charge your body with a fatty acid-filled Krebs cycle.

Medium chain triglycerides are a common additive found in fitness and dieting communities, and it can really have an impact on how effective your ketosis is. Medium chain triglycerides are short, easy to digest fats that are typically found in natural sources but are man-made to act as an additive. Medium chain triglycerides support the quick recovery of muscles during and after a workout, efficient weight loss, and increased energy levels alongside a high concentration of fat. While it isn't necessary to add medium chain triglycerides in order to benefit from just the coffee and butter, it is always important to add as much healthy fat to your carnivore diet as possible in order to balance out your high protein intake and manage your ketosis.

The time-tested recommendation for higher energy levels is, of course, drinking more water, but if you drink too much, you can also begin to experience negative side effects that may lead to an energy slump. Plenty of water tends to flush out your sodium content alongside bodily toxins, which can cause weakness, fatigue, and even fainting. Sprinkling some extra salt on your salmon every once in a while, will help your body maintain its sodium levels so that you can lose weight and if you still feel tired, you can always purchase electrolyte boosters to help rebalance your fluids.

Ingredients for success on a carnivore diet

<u>What You Will Be Eating</u>

Meat, meat, and more meat, and that's no joke. The point of the carnivore diet is to eat only animal sourced foods, this encompasses all of the meat and fish food groups as well as other animal products, namely dairy and eggs. Animal sourced foods are considered to be your classic dairy options, including milk, cheeses, yogurt, and obviously, meat.

One of the most liberating aspects of the carnivore diet is that you don't necessarily have to avoid particularly fatty cuts of meat, although you will want to ensure that your meat is fresh, unprocessed and preferably organic.

Also, when you live as a carnivore you will want to enjoy a diverse diet. Most people that consume a modern western diet are limited in the variety of meat that they eat, often only enjoying steak, chicken brests and bacon, in a typical week. As a carnivore, it's important not only for your body but also your mind to have a diverse array of food that you eat. Organ meats, while not very popular are full of micronutrients and healthy fats, fish contains many of the healthy fats and omega-3 that helps to keep the brain healthy, muscle meats such as chicken, beef, and lamb are packed with protein that your body needs to build and repair. A diversity in your diet will also help you stay on the carnivore diet, as your eating routine won't become monotonous. In short, while you may only be eating animal sourced products, there are so many available that it's important that you retain a diversity in your diet.

So, what do carnivores eat? Chicken thighs are are often popular with carnivores because they have a higher in fat content and a delicious and more robust taste, especially compared to a

34

chicken breast. Similarly, turkey has a very high protein content but doesn't provide the same level of healthy fats, but it can be a welcome change for when you don't feel like eating red meats.

Pork of any style is on the table, from ribs, roasts, and pork belly, to shoulder, and of course everyone's favorite: bacon. Lamb chops and lamb shanks are equally as tasty of dark meat, and a good lamb roast can feed you for days.

When it comes to fish, you are going to want to stick to the healthiest styles you can find; seafood like scallops, mussels, and shrimp, as well as crab, lobster, salmon, trout, and sardines. Anchovies are often high in salt, but they can be great as well.

Beyond meats exclusively, you can incorporate whichever low carbohydrate dairy products you can find; but the catch here is to be wary of the sugar content. Plenty of dairy products, if you'll recall, contain high amounts of processed sugars, and those harmful carbohydrates will affect your ability to reach ketosis. However, you are perfectly able to eat and drink as much milk and cheese as you want if you're mindful of their added carbohydrate content.

Salt is a necessary addition on the carnivore diet, just as it is for any diet. One thing that you will need to decide for yourself is the amount of plant material you allow in your diet in relation to seasoning. Those that are most committed to a carnivore diet will not eat anything that is not animal sourced, others will allow a small amount of plant-based seasoning such as chili or pepper. The idea of allowing some plants in your diet is that it can make the diet easier and more achievable, and the miniscule amount of plant sourced food is trivial, but this will be a decision that you will have to make for yourself. Similarly, you may choose to allow coffee and tea into your diet but as stated before you will need to decide for yourself whether you want to include these into your diet.

Water is essential for the human body, so it's important that you drink plenty of it, but of course not as a fruit juice or soda. One popular beverage for almost all carnivores is bone broth: Not only does bone broth taste great, but it can also be a great way to increase your micronutrient counts as well, as they tend to be packed with calcium, magnesium, iron, and selenium, as well as a whole host of vitamins and micronutrients. What's great about bone broth is that it's an all carnivore hot drink that can be bought from the store, or made cheaply and easily at home; all you have to do is boil the bones, connective tissue, and marrow of either a chicken, cow, pig, or fish, or a combination of all three.

What You Should Avoid

It should come as no shock by now that any ingredient that is not an animal product shouldn't be eaten on a carnivore diet, although as mentioned above many carnivores allow a small amount of coffee or seasoning as an exception.

You will also want to avoid all types of alcohol, as they can be packed with sugars and carbohydrates that will ruin your chances of reaching ketosis. Similarly, any sort of fruit juices that you may enjoy likely won't comply with a carnivore diet.

It's also important to note that you cannot use oils for cooking on a carnivore diet as these will originate from a plant source. Instead, carnivores will often use butter in place of oil for cooking.

Another not so obvious exception to the carnivore diet is processed meats, such as salami. The issue with these products is that despite being made mostly of animal sourced products they contain high amounts of preservatives and often added carbohydrates. For this reason, processed meats such as salamis, sausages, and jerky are not permitted on the carnivore diet.

YOUR PERSONAL CARNIVORE LIFESTYLE

Side effects of low carb diets

You already know that at the beginning of a low carbohydrate diet you may experience withdrawal symptoms that result from a reduction in your sugar intake. This experience is a sign of your body entering a ketogenic state, and is often called the keto flu, this is the most notorious side effect of low carbohydrate diets and has the potential to derail your transition to a carnivorous diet.

Although changing energy levels are normal at the start of any change in your nutrition, a diet that features low carbohydrates will be especially difficult since most of our diet is packed with sugars, even in the fruits and vegetables that we think are healthy. The keto flu presents itself very much like withdrawal, giving you shakiness, sweats, a headache or migraine, and especially if you're overly used to sugar. Common symptoms include fatigue, weakness, irritability, cramps, and digestive distress. While none of these sound like they're enough to put you off a diet, an episode of keto flu symptoms can last for up to five days.

The good news about your carbohydrate flu is that there are plenty of ways to prepare for, and minimize, the potency of its side effects, and there are a few negative side effects you'll want to be familiar with before you begin to eat carnivore. When your body is undergoing digestive distress it is normal that you may experience particularly bad diarrhea in the first few days of eating low carb during your keto flu. There isn't too much you can do to fix this but wait for your body to adjust to the diet, however, some anti-diarrhea may help if this is a severe side effect for you.

One of the strangest side effects of a carnivore diet comes when you reach full ketosis and develop horrible bad breath. With a smell that is similar to acetone, or nail polish remover, the bad breath associated with keto diets is actually a good sign. If you'll recall, acetone is one of the three ketone components that make up a ketone body. When you reach ketosis and begin to function solely off the energy you get from ketones, some of that acetone finds its way into your breath. The easiest fix for this side effect is simply a stick of gum or a breath mint.

Minimizing your symptoms

Combatting the keto flu is one of the best ways to make sure that you last into the fat burning stages of ketosis on your carnivore diet. One of the best ways to reduce the impact of carbohydrate withdrawals is to set aside two to three weeks before your carnivore diet begins to properly ween yourself off of addictive glucose sugars.

The western diet is high in sugars both in what we eat and what we drink, so start with your daily beverage consumption and eliminate all sugary sodas, juices, and anything essentially that isn't water. This might be hard for the first few days, but this will give your system the opportunity to get used to a lower level of carbohydrate intake before eliminating carbs completely. As mentioned earlier if you want something tasty to drink, you can always have a mug of tea, coffee, or bone broth.

If you drink more than one soda a day or put sugar in your coffee or tea, begin by simply reducing your intake by half at first and then reduce further.

Drinking water is another essential part of preparing your body for a carnivore diet, not only will this help to keep you hydrated, but it will also help to reduce the amount of plant toxins in your body.

Hunger control, carnivore style

Hunger pangs can be one of the most difficult symptoms to struggle through on a new diet. Hunger pangs are caused by the hormone ghrelin, but the tricky thing about hunger pangs is that most of our bodies aren't actually lacking food, we are lacking something else, but our bodies can become confused and things such as dehydration or high blood sugar can lead to a hungry stomach that doesn't actually need food.

On the carnivore diet, you'll be supplying your body with only healthy fats in order to stimulate fat catabolism. When you eat a diet that is high in processed sugars and artificial ingredients, your body gets used to large spikes in your blood sugar that develop similar insulin resistance and type 2 diabetes.

If your bloodstream is packed with too much glucose, you develop insulin resistance, and then your cells do not absorb sugar for energy. You have plenty of calories, and plenty of sugar, available for use, but it can't get to where it needs to be, and so you experience hunger pangs.

Similarly, when you're dehydrated, your body will crave foods like fruit or candy that taste sweet which we associate with quenching our thirst. Hunger pangs can be incredibly misleading, and when you're operating on a fully carnivorous diet, you should barely have any. Eating on fats and proteins consistently allows your digestion to regulate and settle on one consistent food source, and we all know how important it is for our bodies to remain balanced. Once your insulin levels reregulate and your blood sugar goes down, your body can manage your hunger pangs by searching in your already robust supply of glucose. Just like that, you'll get hungrier less often, and usually carnivores will consume fewer meals.

Your carnivore transition

Once you've properly primed your body to begin eating a carnivore diet, you are going to notice certain changes throughout your first week that, while they differ from person to person, are largely the same across the board. If you took the time to ween yourself off of carbohydrates before your carnivore diet began, you probably only felt flu-like symptoms for the first three days.

On day four, it is most likely that your digestion will begin to re-regulate, and you should have noticed your hunger pangs getting more and more faint. This is the point at which most people feel comfortable adding in a bulletproof coffee because the effects will be ten-fold on your already slowly recovering body. If you haven't yet experienced an easing in your headaches, don't worry. Dehydration can occur throughout the first four days as your digestion struggles to keep up with inflammation, irritation, and proper water absorption.

By day ten, you should feel the best you have ever felt. Your sleeping schedule should have normalized, your brain fog will have cleared, and you should have entered into full ketosis.

Speaking of brain fog, your cognitive function by day ten should be better than you've known in years. Ketones are a powerful source, and you shouldn't be surprised if you're more focused, positive, and consistent in output. During this time, you will also find your energy at the gym has increased, and this is the best time to re-integrate high intensity interval training and weightlifting into your regime. At this point, your carnivore diet is up and running, and you shouldn't be experiencing any more negative side effects.

Many individuals who start a carnivore diet, or any low carb diet, chose to keep a food journal throughout their first few days or weeks, of dieting. However, there are a few benefits and drawbacks to journaling so early. The best time to start really keeping track of your nutrition is by day ten when you're feeling at your best and can cut out all the excess helpers you used to get you through the carb flu.

It's recommended to start with an accurate food journal, in the beginning, adding in your caffeine and butter, if you include it, and whatever excess fat intake you needed to keep yourself going.

Keeping exact track of your macronutrients in your prime state of ketosis will help keep you there. A food journal can also help you diagnose problems if you start to find that you aren't losing as much weight eating only meat as you thought. Sometimes, you might need to cut back on the dairy, the protein, or the overall caloric amount that you're taking in in order to maximize weight loss on a carnivore diet.

Meal prepping your carnivore diet

Meal preparation has been a staple in the fitness and body building communities for a long time, because of its easy, helpful, and organized style. Diets can be hard to stick to if you are running around between the gym, work, home, and whatever you do in your free time. If you find yourself hungry in the middle of the day without a proper snack, it can be a huge energy drain to go hungry while you wait for your next healthy meal or snack. Preparing your meals and snacks ahead of time and packaging them up will help you better track what you are eating, how much you are eating, and when you are eating.

The idea behind meal prepping is that each weekend before you begin your work week, you will take the time to prepare portioned out entrees for either lunch, dinner, or both that can be refrigerated and heated up for nutrition on command. Most meal preppers do their grocery shopping and cooking on Sundays to make sure that their meals are as fresh as possible for the week ahead. When it comes to meal prepping specifically for a carnivore diet, we'll go over a few cooking tricks in the recipe section, but usually you'll want to prepare between three and four portions of each entrée. Once you have each portion separated out evenly in Tupperware, make sure to use masking tape and a sharpie to write the date you cooked each one. Many meals can be frozen and stored for a long time, so by having a few meals frozen and ready, you will always have a choice of fresh carnivore meals to choose from, which will help to keep you motivated and your diet diverse.

Meal prep is also highly beneficial for those of you that want to track your macronutrients in order to make sure you're getting the right portions of fat and protein. If you don't already use MyFitnessPal or a similar fitness tracker, you can utilize an online calculator to enter the amount of each ingredient in the dish and the weight of the dish to estimate its nutritional content including the protein content and fat content of each meal.

It's likely that you don't eat every meal at home, and typically, most carnivores won't pre-prepare a meal for their Thursday or Friday in case they have exciting weekend plans with friends. But for a carnivore diet, it can be very difficult to attempt to eat at a restaurant. Let's look at some of the best ways to make use of your non-meal prep days so that you can stay social while you eat carnivore.

Eating a carnivore diet for travelling and vacation

When you aren't at home, it can be a bit more difficult to eat a healthy carnivore diet that is high in unprocessed meats and low carbohydrate dairy. However, when you're travelling or spending the holidays with non-carnivorous eaters, there are a few easy changes you can make. When you're travelling it can be especially difficult to control the food you ingest when you have not prepared it yourself.

During breakfast, you can make easy egg-based switches that will account for a decent amount of your 35% protein before breakfast. Choosing items like omelets filled with natural cheeses and avoiding pastry items will fill you up on proteins that won't have you feeling hungry around mid-morning. Breakfast is also a great place to build up your healthy fats with meats like ham and bacon that are available at almost any buffet, even continental hotel spreads. Coffee is your best friend while you are away from a constant source of meat-based nutrition, and if you can't find another decent snack around lunchtime, it can be useful to keep some meat snacks to keep in your hotel fridge.

One of the most important skills you can develop while eating a carnivore diet is learning to pick up healthy meat and animal sourced snacks that don't require a lot of cooking. Pre-packaged cheeses can also fit in easily accessible places and won't break your carnivore diet. When you're eating for a holiday meal at someone else's home, you'll want to make sure that you make preparations in advance.

If you're eating with friends and family, most of the time, no one will argue if you offer to bring something – be it a side dish, appetizer, or entrée. If you plan ahead and prepare your own entrees to share that will be delicious and nutritious for you, and also a kind gesture for your loved ones, you can keep with your diet and still celebrate socially. Plenty of traditional holiday recipes can be adapted to be either vegan or vegetarian, and if you can adapt a dish to have no meat, you can adapt a dish to have no vegetables. If you aren't able to bring your own dishes to a holiday meal, it's just as easy to survey your options and make a decision from what is available. Party platters will often be packed with cubed cheeses and skewed meats.

Also, don't forget about the importance of eggs for more than just breakfast. You can hard boil a protein filled egg snack for a boost of energy or salt and pepper devilled eggs.

How to sustain a social diet

With a limited range of ingredients available for you to consume while eating a carnivore diet, it is no surprise that many carnivore dieters find it difficult to eat with friends, out at a restaurant, or at someone else's house. Diets by themselves tend to be restricting, but there are a few great tips and tricks that can allow you to be social and still maintain a meat-only carnivorous diet. Though it may give you extra work before a fun dinner party, checking the menu of a restaurant you'll be eating at, that is if you didn't pick the venue, will help you be better prepared for what healthy, carnivorous options they have available. In the event that your friends trust you to pick the place, it's always a good idea to have an arsenal of great carnivore-friendly restaurants at the ready. Also don't be afraid to make a choice where you know you won't be able to eat the entire dish; for example, if you order steak and vegetables, it's perfectly fine to eat the steak and not the vegetables, and you can always ask your server if there is an substation that can be made.

Barbecue places, grills, and culinary kitchens will typically offer plenty of meat-friendly options. You should note that a steakhouse is the best establishment to visit on a carnivore diet. Don't be afraid to make substitutions either when it comes to ordering for a carnivore diet at a restaurant. Plenty of establishments will offer sides of bacon, a steak without the potatoes or vegetables, or shrimp and scallops on their own. Kitchen staff are always happy to help if you chose to cut out ingredients, and don't be afraid to order a steak with exactly what you want – only salt and pepper. If you have a hankering for meat that isn't your regular porterhouse, any barbecue joints will satisfy your cravings as long as you avoid the sauce. Dry brisket cooked well is just as tasty as brisket covered in sugary barbecue sauce.

FREQUENTLY ASKED CARNIVORE DIET QUESTIONS

Is the carnivore diet safe?

The carnivore diet, like any diet, is safe and healthy as long as you are responsible, listen to your body, and follow good advice. Eating only meat might sound unconventional, but as discussed earlier in the book, the human body is able to access all of the micro and macronutrients that it requires solely from meat. The basis of the carnivore diet is similar to the benefits enjoyed by those on a ketogenic diet, and many ketogenic dieters also cut out fruits and certain starchy vegetables; a carnivorous diet eliminates harmful carbohydrate sugars to an extreme level for maximized weight loss, muscles gains, and mental clarity.

<u>Do you eat any vegetables on the carnivore diet?</u>

No. On the carnivore diet, you will eat only meat and low carbohydrate animal sourced products. Animal sourced products can be anything from milk and dairy to cheese and eggs, but you should always make sure that if your ingredients are whole, unprocessed, and still contain a proper nutritional balance. Look for low carbohydrate dairy products that won't spike your blood sugar in order to keep your diet balanced without vegetable fiber to slow down your digestion.

<u>How much weight will I lose on a carnivore diet?</u>

The carnivore diet aims to help you reach a healthy weight by rewiring your body to breakdown the fat that's already present in your body, this process will help you excess weight without having to do input extra effort at the gym.

<u>What's the best way to keep chicken interesting?</u>

Chicken is a weightlifter's favorite source of protein, but with only salt and pepper as seasonings allowed on a carnivore diet, it can be hard to spice up relatively bland meat. While we'll discuss cooking techniques specific to meat in the next section, tossing a chicken breast on the grill will give you a nice added chargrilled flavor without compromising your carnivore diet. Similarly, make sure that you take advantage of the whole of the animal, including the wings, legs, thighs, skin, and livers. This is a great way to add variety to your regime as well as to your nutritional intake.

How much protein do you eat on a carnivore diet?

Typical carnivore diets don't dictate a specific ratio of protein to fat, but nutritionists tend to recommend that you eat around 65% fat and 35% protein on a diet that is entirely devoid of carbohydrates. While you are welcome to adjust this figure up and down accordingly based on your personal preferences, you should be able to reach ketosis and maintain a healthy carnivore diet by keeping close to this ratio.

Should I stay away from cuts of meat that are particularly fatty?

Absolutely, not. Fatty cuts of meat and entirely fine to eat on a carnivore diet, and in fact, the more natural animal fat you can consume that hasn't been processed, the better. Ribs tend to contain the highest concentration of natural fat, which makes sense for where they're located on the body. However, you can't go wrong with adding in more healthy whole fats to a diet that needs 65%.

Can you survive on an all meat diet?

Yes, and more than that you can thrive. Humans have survived on meat and animal sourced foods for thousands of years, and there's no reason why we shouldn't be able to do so in the modern world. The carnivore diet is designed to eliminate all the unhealthy processed sugars that are damaging your health and replace them with natural, animal sourced foods.

With rising rates of heart disease and obesity, a more accurate question would be; can you survive on a modern western diet?

How do I start eating an all-meat diet?

The short answer is to just stop eating anything that isn't meat. The better and slightly longer answer is that you should first understand the effects that eating an all-meat diet will have, and then beginning to prepare for a transition. As mentioned earlier in this book, creating a routine makes the diet much easier to handle, and so the more that you a prepare before beginning the easier it will be.

Finally, adjusting to an all meat diet can come with some withdrawal symptoms and digestive distress, and for that reason it's important that you understand that this is a normal part of the carnivore diet and is only temporary.

<u>Can you have dairy on a carnivore diet?</u>

Yes, dairy is absolutely allowed on a carnivore diet. Dairy is considered an animal sourced food, which means that it comes from an animal and not from a plant.

The issue that some carnivores have with diary is that it milk contains a sugar called lactose, and while lactose is considered a sugar unless very large quantities are ingested this is unlikely to have a significantly detrimental effect on your carnivore diet. Too much of anything is bad for you, but dairy is an ingredient whose nutritional value has been vastly underrated. When you're eating a diet rich in whole, healthy fats, animal milk, butter, and creams are one of the best ways to incorporate them into your diet.

Can you drink alcohol on the carnivore diet?

Alcohol is almost never condoned as part of any sort of nutritional plan and will always do harm to your body in a way that most fitness programs do not condone. Specifically, for your carnivore diet, alcohol contains too much sugar to be fit for supporting ketosis. The only beverages that you are allowed to consume while eating a carnivore diet are water, coffee, tea, and bone broth.

Isn't red meat bad for your health?

Red meat is incredibly healthy when it is found in its natural unprocessed state. Humans have been consuming vast quantities of red meat for thousand or years without any side effects, and it is not surprising that individuals who eat carnivore diets today also tend to show no adverse side effects. Unprocessed red meat is packed with essential micronutrients like vitamin B12, antioxidants, selenium, zinc, and iron.

Will I lose muscle tone on a low carb diet?

The Atkin's diet, the keto diet, paleo diet, and all your other low carbohydrate regimes tend to scare people away because of their inability to sustain large and significant gains.

Carbohydrates are supposedly what our bodies need to build muscles, but you can use your ketone body fuel and fatty acids to make just as much progress in the gym. On a carnivore diet, you'll be eating almost 35% of your diet in protein.

<u>Can I still lift weights on the carnivore diet?</u>

Once you reach ketosis, the energy your body can harvest from ketone bodies will give you all the power you need to continue weightlifting. While you might have to take a few days off from your regime at the beginning of your diet, after you adjust to eating only meats, your energy and strength will be double what it was before. Take things slowly as you adjust to your new energy levels, and make sure to listen to your body as your workout. In between lifting sessions be sure to work on strengthening exercises as well as flexibility in order to stay limber without stressing yourself out during a transition period.

RECIPES AND COOKING GUIDE

Overview of preparation techniques

The main ways that you'll be preparing your meats depend on the cut and style of the meat itself, as well as the overall outcome that you're looking for. Meat and animal products almost always need to be cooked well to kill off any bacteria on their surface, but there are ways that you can use cooking to maximize the flavor of your food. You can always use your oven if you don't want to grill, and the metal racks will offer you extra space to lay out long cuts. In the backyard, a smoker grill can lend delicious thick flavor to your steaks without sucking out their moisture. Adding in charcoal pellets to your outdoor grill will allow you to smoke your meats with new flavors, while any sort of wood like hickory can also add a level of nuance that will have you wondering why you ever used so much barbecue sauce. When it comes to cuts of meat, you already know that fatty cuts are entirely on the menu, but you'll want to make sure to cook these in a cast iron skillet to really lock in the fatty oils that the meat expels during cooking.

CARNIVORE BREAKFASTS

CLASSIC BACON AND EGGS

INGREDIENTS:

½ tbsp full-fat animal butter

4 large eggs

2 thick cut strips of bacon

2 thick cut cubes of pork belly

Sea salt and black pepper to preference

METHOD:

When it comes to cooking on your carnivore diet, it's a great idea to take advantage of all the animal fat possible that cooks off from the heat. In a medium skillet warmed with your low carb, full-fat animal butter, cook your bacon halfway. Add in the pork belly cuts and cook until both are desirably crispy. Remove the bacon and cook your eggs sunny side up in the bacon grease until your yolk is your preferred texture. Season with sea salt and black pepper.

GRILLED FLANK STANK WITH PEPPER EGGS

INGREDIENTS:

3 pounds (lbs.) of flank steak

1 tbsp room-temperature animal butter

1 tsp sea salt

1 tsp ground black pepper

4 large eggs

METHOD:

The night before you cook this meal, rub your flank stank on either side with the room-temperature animal butter and your sea salt and ground black pepper. Marinate the steak in your refrigerator overnight and grill the next morning either on a barbecue grill or on a stovetop grill. Cook your eggs however you'd like and serve with the steak on top of the eggs. Sea salt and pepper to preference.

CHICKEN BREAKFAST TOSTADAS

INGREDIENTS:

2 cups white cheddar cheese

2 oz cooked and shredded chicken

1 tbsp full-fat animal butter

½ cup ground chorizo sausage

¼ cup of parmesan

Sea salt and black pepper to preference

METHOD:

While your oven preheats to 375°F, lay out a baking tray with aluminum foil greased in animal butter. After making small one-inch rounds of white cheddar cheese, bake your cheese tostada bases in the oven until they're brown and crispy, about 5 minutes. As the cheese rounds cook, warm a medium skillet over medium heat with your tablespoon of full-fat animal butter. Cook your chorizo until moist and brown, and then cook one full room temperature chicken breast until you can pull it apart with two forks. Once your cheese rounds are crispy, let them cool, and then plate with chicken, chorizo, and garnish with parmesan cheese.

CARNIVORE LEGENDARY BREAKFAST PIZZA

INGREDIENTS:

8-10 large eggs

½ cups ground chorizo sausage

¼ cups shredded American cheese

¼ cups goat cheese

Ground black pepper to preference

METHOD:

In a medium bowl, whisk together your eggs so that the yolks and whites combine to create a uniform mixture. Pour the egg mixture into a non-stick pie pan greased with animal butter and bake in a 350°F oven until solid but not brown, the texture of a quiche. Meanwhile, heat another tablespoon of animal butter in a medium skillet and cook your chorizo sausage until brown and moist. Layer your pizza egg crust first, then chorizo sausage, topped with goat cheese and black pepper to taste.

POACHED EGG AND HAM CARNIVORE BENEDICT

CARNIVORE FAUX HOLLANDAISE:

3 large eggs

¼ tsp sea salt

¼ tsp ground black pepper

½ cups full-fat animal butter

1 tbsp lemon extract (purely chemical, no carbohydrates added)

ENTRéE:

2 large eggs

2 oz of sliced ham, unprocessed

Sea salt and black pepper to preference

METHOD:

In a blender, combine your sea salt, black pepper, lemon extract, and egg yolks while you melt the animal butter in a small skillet over medium heat. Allow the blender to run at a low speed, and simultaneously pour in the hot animal butter until the two mixtures are combined in the blender. As the hollandaise thickens, you can begin to poach your eggs in an electronic poacher. Add your ham slices to the warmed butter in your skillet and cook until brown and crispy. Serve together and garnish with your hollandaise sauce.

CARNIVORE LUNCHES

BACON-WRAPPED CARNIVORE MEATLOAF

INGREDIENTS:

1 tbsp full-fat animal butter

1½ lb. ground beef

1 cup shredded cheddar cheese

½ cups of parmesan cheese

2 egg yolks

1 egg white

6 – 8 slices of regular cut bacon

Sea salt and black pepper to preference

METHOD:

While your oven preheats to 400*F, use a large bowl to mix together your ground beef, egg yolks, and white, sea salt, black pepper, parmesan, and cheddar into a large meatloaf shape. Once you have greased an oven-safe glass baking dish with more animal butter, place the bacon strips with their bottom tips already in the dish. Once you've placed your meatloaf, fold the bacon strips over the loaf and cook until each slice is crispy – approximately 1 hour. If your bacon starts to burn sooner than 1 hour in, wrap your dish in aluminum foil.

TASTY CARNIVORE CHEESE TACOS

INGREDIENTS:

2½ cups shredded cheddar cheese

1 lb. ground beef

6 – 8 large tiger prawns, peeled and veined

Sea salt and black pepper to preference

METHOD:

Once you have preheated your oven to 375°F, lay out ½" tall circles of shredded cheddar cheese like cookie dough on a baking sheet that you've greased with animal butter. Keeping an eye on the rounds, cook your cheesy until just barely crispy – about 5 minutes. Meanwhile, in a warm skillet lined with animal butter, cook your ground beef seasoned with sea salt and pepper until brown throughout. In the same skillet once you've removed the beef, cook your tiger shrimp until they are pink but not overly white in color. Once your taco cheese rounds are crispy, transfer them to a metal taco base or to a taco mold to cool. Layer each cheese taco with ground beef and shrimp to top.

OPEN-FACE TURKEY BACON SANDWICH

INGREDIENTS:

1 lb. ground turkey meat

1 tbsp of animal butter

3 slices of thin cute hickory-smoked bacon

½ cups of white cheddar cheese

METHOD:

While you warm a medium skillet with animal butter, combine your ground turkey meat and white cheddar cheese in a bowl, kneading with your hands to form small sliders patties. Once your pan has warmed, cook each slice of bacon until its desired crispness and set aside. In the still-hot pan with bacon grease, cook your turkey sliders until they are tender but not too soft in the middle, checking for pinkness if necessary. Layer each slider with two half-slices of crispy bacon for a delicious carnivore BLT without the LT.

SLOW-COOKED SOUTHERN BEEF BRISKET

INGREDIENTS:

2 lb. flat cut beef brisket, fat untrimmed

1 tsp of sea salt

1 tsp teaspoons of ground black pepper

3 tbsp full-fat animal butter

METHOD:

While your oven preheats to 350°F, pat your brisket strips with your ground black pepper. Over the stove, heat a large skillet over medium to high heat with the animal butter. Once your butter has melted, brown each brisket strip in the butter, waiting for each side to crisp and turn golden – about 7 minutes. Garnish with sea salt to taste and let rest for 5 minutes.

BLACKENED SALMON

INGREDIENTS:

2 salmon fillets, approximately 4oz each

2 tsp of sea salt

2 tsp ground black pepper

½ cup full-fat melted animal butter

METHOD

Warm a large skillet over the stove with 0.25 cups of butter melting in the bottom. While your skillet warms, mix together your salt and pepper with the other 0.25 cups of melted butter. Once you have glazed each side of your salmon fillets with butter, cook them until the fish begins to flake in pink chunks. Let rest for 2 minutes and then serve.

HOMEMADE CHARCUTERIE PLATE

INGREDIENTS:

4 strips of full-fat prosciutto

4 strips of Sopressata salami

4 strips of smoked salmon

1oz goats' cheese

1oz of Havarti

1oz of brie

METHOD:

A charcuterie plate might sound like something that you would only eat a high-class restaurant, but discount cheese blocks and charcuterie slices that are high in fatty meats will supply you with plenty of fats and proteins to support ketosis. And, it's a great way to fill up on lunch by eating smaller, more targeted snacks with a variety of flavor profiles. Because you can't eat crackers or grains alongside your charcuterie boards, you should aim to eat twice as much meat per slice of cheese to balance your flavors. Slice your cheeses in thing rectangles when you can, and pair them with 2" slices of charcuterie meat for the perfect high-fat, full-meat animal sourced lunch.

LOBSTER TAILS WITH ANIMAL BUTTER

INGREDIENTS:

2 lobster tails, 3-5oz each

¼ tsp ground black pepper

1 ½ tbsp melted full-fat animal butter

¼ tsp sea salt

METHOD:

In order to properly cut your lobster tails, point the tip of your kitchen scissor upwards through the curved edge of the top of the lobster tail when sat on a plate facing downwards. Once you've cut through the shell to the tail, turn the lobster over and crack the crustacean's ribs down the center. After removing the shell with your thumbs and fingers, lift the lobster meat out of the shell. Word to the wise – lobster tails can be sharp, so go slowly with minimal pressure. Once you have extracted the lobster meat, cook each tail on the middle rack of your oven preheated to a strong 5 hundred-degree broil. Add a cube of animal butter to each tail, and broil until the meat is at least 145°F. Cool for 10 minutes, then serve.

SAVORY BAKED CHICKEN THIGHS

INGREDIENTS:

2 chicken thighs

½ tsp of sea salt

1½ tsp ground black pepper

1 tbsp full-fat animal fat

METHOD:

In a clean oven-safe glass baking dish, use melted animal butter to create a non-stick layer. After the dish is ready, preheat your oven to 375°F. Once you have rubbed each chicken thigh thoroughly with salt and pepper, bake for thirty minutes or until the chicken juices run clear – each thigh should reach 165°F internally before cooling. Garnish with 0.25 cups of parmesan cheese for taste.

BISON MEATBALLS

INGREDIENTS:

2 lb. organically sourced bison chuck

2 tbsp full-fat animal butter

2½ tbsp non-flavored protein powder, or more for a thicker consistency

3 egg yolks

METHOD:

In a medium bowl, combine your bison chuck with melted animal butter, protein powder, and egg yolks. While your oven preheats to 375°F, form bison meatballs that are each the size of a one-inch golf ball. Cook your bison meatballs on an aluminum foil tray greased with animal butter for at least twenty minutes, or until browned and crispy.

TROUT WITH PROVOLONE AND PINK PEPPERCORNS

INGREDIENTS:

4oz fillet of wild-caught trout

½ cup shredded provolone cheese

¼ tsp ground pink peppercorns

1 tbsp full-fat animal butter

METHOD:

In a medium skillet over melted full-fat animal butter, cook your trout piece skin-down for at least twenty minutes until the fish on top is flaky. Once you have achieved your desired consistency, remove the trout from the heat and season with sea salt and ground pink peppercorns. Garnish with shredded provolone cheese and rest for 2 minutes before serving. Be sure to avoid ingesting the skin.

CARNIVORE DINNERS

SLOW-COOKER NO-VEGGIE CHILI

INGREDIENTS:

2oz chicken breast, cooked and shredded

½ lb. ground beef

½ lb. ground turkey

2 cups cubed pork belly

8-10 cups of bone broth

1 cup mozzarella cheese

½ cup yellow cheddar cheese

Sea salt and black pepper to preference

METHOD:

To make your bone broth, boil together with the bones, connective tissues, and marrow of either chicken, pork, beef, or all three, simmering for more than 24 hours if your mixture includes more red meat bones than chicken bones, but only 24 hours if you chose to cook only chicken.

After a maximum of forty-eight hours, strain your broth. In a large slow cooker set to medium, add in your bone broth, turkey, pork belly, chicken, and your cheeses. Leave to cook for at least 6 hours, stirring if you can. After 6 hours, let cool and garnish with parmesan cheese.

CARNIVORE SURF AND TURF

INGREDIENTS:

1 tbsp melted full-fat animal butter

¼ tsp fresh ground pepper

¼ tsp of sea salt

4oz filet mignon steak

10 – 12 large prawns, peeled and veined

METHOD:

In a large bowl, combine all your shrimp with the sea salt and pepper and then cover to refrigerate for at least fifteen minutes. With your grill turned up to medium or high heat depending on your personal preference, cook your steak until as tough or tender as you wish. Once your steak has finished, cook your shrimp either on skewers or in an aluminum foil boat until pink but not solidly white. Dress with more sea salt and pepper to taste.

DUCK CARNIVORE CONFIT

INGREDIENTS:

4 cups duck fat

½ tsp sea salt

1½ tsp ground black pepper

½ tsp black peppercorns

2 trimmed and reserved duck legs (thighs attached)

METHOD:

12 hours before your meal, season each duck leg and thigh with your sea salt and ground black pepper before laying each leg skin side down in an oven-safe glass container with your duck fat already in the bottom. Once the legs and thighs have refrigerated for 12 hours, preheat your oven to 300°F before rinsing each leg in cold water. Once the legs are dry (you can dry them with paper towels), dress the legs in more duck fat and leave them to cook, covered, for 2½-3 hours. Once the duck meat is supple and falling off the bone, serve.

CRISPY RIBEYE ROAST

INGREDIENTS:

16oz ounce ribeye steak, approximately 1.5" thick

½ tsp sea salt

¼ tsp ground black pepper

2½ tbsp full-fat animal butter

METHOD:

While you preheat your oven to 500°F, warm a large cast iron skillet over the stove on high heat with your 2½ tablespoons of animal butter. Once the butter has melted, sear your ribeye steak on either side for no more than thirty seconds. Making sure to spoon hot butter over the steak as you do this, allow the ribeye to rest for 5 minutes in the oven. After another 5 minutes resting in the oven, you're ready to serve.

BACON-WRAPPED SCALLOPS WITH BUTTER SAUCE

INGREDIENTS:

4 scallops, approximately 1oz each

4 strips of thick cut fatty bacon

2 tbsp full-fat animal butter

2 tsp sea salt

2 tsp of black ground pepper

4 egg yolks

METHOD:

In a blender, combine your sea salt, ground black pepper, and eggs yolks and blend. While your blender works, warm a large cast iron skillet over medium to high heat. Once your skillet is hot, crisp the bacon in its own fat until the sides are opaque in color, but not yet crispy – each piece should be relatively flaccid. Remove the bacon at this point and add 1 tbsp of animal butter. Turn the blender off and let your butter sauce rest. Once the butter has begun to bubble, sauté your scallops so that each side is seared and crispy brown, spending no longer than 45 seconds on each flat circular side, and twenty seconds to sear each round vector in a circle along the sides. Once your scallops are cooked, remove the skillet from heat and use tongs to wrap each scallop in the limp bacon. Place the cast iron skillet into an oven preheated to 450°F, and broil for 5 minutes, watching for early browning. Remove the bacon-wrapped scallops once they crisp, and dress with room temperature butter sauce once plated.

PORK TENDERLOIN

INGREDIENTS:

3 tbsp full-fat animal butter

1 lb. pork tenderloin

1 tsp sea salt

1 tsp ground black pepper

Parmesan for garnish

METHOD:

In a medium frying pan or cast-iron skillet containing melted full-fat animal butter, lay your pork tenderloin log in the center of the pan with your tongs ready. Keeping watch over your tenderloin, turn the log once each side has cooked enough to color and crisp on the outside, but not yet brown the rare pink in the center. Once each of your sides has been seared to your liking (and the meat has reached at least 145°F internally), allow the tenderloin to rest before cutting into 1-1½" disks and serving with more butter, salt, and pepper to preference. Garnish with parmesan if desired.

CARNIVORE CLASSIC LAMB CHOPS

INGREDIENTS:

5 tbsp melted full-fat animal butter

1½ tsp sea salt

1½ tsp ground black pepper

2 large lamb chops

METHOD:

In a small bowl while your grill warms up, combine your full-fat animal butter, sea salt, and pepper in a small bowl and mix. Using a basting brush, glaze each lamb chop with the mixture. Grill each lamb chop over medium to high heat for up to 4 minutes for a tender medium rare, measuring the internal temperature to ensure the meat reaches at least 140°F. Rest the chops for 10 minutes, then serve.

FULL AT-HOME ROTISSERIE CHICKEN

INGREDIENTS:

3 lb. whole raw chicken

¼ cup full-fat melted animal butter

1 tsp sea salt

1 tsp ground black pepper

METHOD:

Before you begin to cook, combine your full-fat animal butter, sea salt, and pepper in a small bowl, and mix until even. Once your rotisserie or rotating spit is hot enough, turn your whole chicken after seasoning all over with 1 tsp salt. Once the skin of the chicken begins to moisten, glaze with more melted animal butter and grill on medium heat, basting the entire chicken with animal butter every twenty minutes. After an hour and a half, or until the chicken is brown and at 180°F, remove and let stand for at least fifteen minutes.

CARNIVORE ORGAN BLOOD SAUSAGE

INGREDIENTS:

2 cups pure pork blood

½ lb. pork fat

1 lb. duck fat, either liquid or hardened

1 tbsp fresh ground pepper

2½ tbsp sea salt

½ lb. pure pork fat, frozen

15 feet of sausage casing

METHOD:

Begin by sectioning off your pork fat based on sharp knife cuts through room-temperature pieces – you should end up with cubes that can be effectively frozen. Repeat the same process with your duck lard, and then dump each pork cube into a plastic bag and leave to harden in the freezer. While your pork fat freezes, mix the seal salt and ground pepper. Once you have cut rectangles out of the pork and fat, mix your meats in with your seasonings. Making sure to combine everything thoroughly and evenly, chill the entire mixture in the refrigerator for at least 2 hours. Once the temperature has reached close to freezing, remove it and place in a mixer. Slowly add in the pork blood to the meat and fat, blending until creamy and thick. Place your hog sausage casing in a bowl of warm water and place the blood mixture back in the freezer. Meanwhile, bring a second pot to a steaming simmer, but not quite a boil, and fill a large bowl with ice water. Fill your sausage casings with no warmer than 35°F blood sausage mixture. Then, boil each sausage in the warm water for fifteen minutes before blitzing with cold.

CHICKEN LIVER PATE

INGREDIENTS:

3 cups room-temperature water

¾ cup full-fat animal butter

¼ tsp ground black pepper

½ tsp of sea salt

1½ lb. chicken liver

METHOD:

Over medium heat, bring a medium-sized saucepan to medium or high heat with ¼ cup of full-fat animal butter to prevent sticking. Add your water and livers until the mixture reaches a boil, and then cover while reducing to low heat. Once the liquid mixture turns brown, drain the mixtures of throw away any thicker, chunkier sections of the filtered-out liver. Combine your softened saucepan ingredients together in a food processor or blender and blitz until smooth. You can serve either hot or cold, but most classical liver pates are served chilled in a rectangular bread-baking tin to create smooth, even sandwich slices.

ONE-WEEK CARNIVORE MEAL PLAN

To begin your one-week carnivore diet, we're going to start with the shopping ingredients that you'll need to prepare your meals in advance on Saturday or Sunday. Ideally, you'll prepare your meals on Sunday to maximize their freshness, Saturday will also work just fine. It's an added bonus that your ingredient list is already fairly limited, so you won't need to spend too much of your day at the shops. When you go grocery shopping on a carnivore diet, you'll want to avoid the produce section entirely, as well as any other sections besides seafood, the deli, and dairy.

For this one-week plan, you will be cooking two lunch meals and two dinner meals together on the weekend day of your choice, as well as preparing small carnivorous snacks to keep with you throughout the week. Breakfast is a little bit trickier, as it usually needs to be made fresh, but with easy-to-cook ingredients like eggs and bacon, each of these breakfast recipes will take under twenty minutes to cook. To maximize your time cooking breakfast each week, pick only two meals to alternate between each day. If you're ready to start your first week on a carnivore diet, let's take a look at what your weekend cooking schedule should look like.

<u>Shopping list</u>

12 lb. flank steak

4 lb. lean fat-free beef

4 lb. of bison chuck

16 slices of thick cut bacon

2½ lb. pork belly 4 lb. of pork tenderloin

2 large lamb chops

3 4oz salmon fillets

30 large eggs

3 lb. tbsp full-fat animal butter

8oz grated fresh parmesan

Sea salt

Black pepper

<u>Meal Prep Cooking Steps</u>

Begin by marinating your flank steaks for 12 hours, overnight, the day before you begin meal-prepping. Marinate each steak in full-fat animal butter, sea salt, and black pepper before wrapping them in a plastic bag and letting sit in the fridge.

<u>Lunches:</u>

Line a large skillet with full-fat animal butter and warm over the stove. While your butter melts, combine the bison chuck, melted animal butter, protein powder, and eggs yolks in a medium bowl. Mix together thoroughly and set aside – refrigeration helps the mixture maintain its consistency, so feel free to cover and let cool. Preheat your oven to 180°F. Once your butter begins to bubble, mix together another ¼ cup of melted butter with your sea salt and pepper, and brush your salmon fillets. Cook each side for approximately 5 minutes, or until the fish flakes. Remove from heat and let stand. Taking the cooled bison chuck mixture, form one-inch balls and place on an aluminum foil tray greased with animal butter. Bake for at least twenty minutes, or until desirably brown. Let cool and store your six lunch meals in Tupperware.

<u>Dinners:</u>

Begin by warming up your grill, and as this happens, combine in a small bowl your full-fat animal butter, sea salt, and ground black pepper. Use a basting brush to glaze each lamb chop, then grill for at least 4 minutes on either side or until the internal temperature of the lamb reaches 140°F. After finishing the first chop, set a large cast iron skillet on the stove with one tablespoon of animal butter melting in the bottom. Once you've finished your second chop, the butter should be bubbling. Start the third chop and place your pork tenderloin log in the center of your skillet with tongs. Keeping watch over your lamb chop, slowly rotate the pork tenderloin until each long side is browned and cooked but the center remains pink. Leave your lamb chops to rest and garnish with sea salt and black pepper. Once your tenderloin has finished, allow it to rest for at least 5 minutes before cutting into 1½" medallions. Garnish with melted butter, sea salt, and pepper. Parmesan can be added for taste, but only on the day, you eat your meal. Cheese doesn't always save well in Tupperware. Package your six dinners and keep in the freezer to save fridge space.

<u>Snack Steps:</u>

Wrap your lean cut of beef in plastic wrap and place it in the freezer for up to two hours. While you wait, fill a large pot with cold water so that the level just covers the top of your eggs. Bring the water to a rolling boil, then cover the pot, remove from heat, and let sit for 10 minutes. With a sharp knife, slice thin, even slices until you've cut all pounds. Combine the melted butter, sea salt, and pepper and mix until combined. In a large bowl, combine the butter marinade and the beef slice, and cover while refrigerating for up to 24 hours. Drain and dry the beef slices, then, in a 300°F oven, blitz the slices while they lay over your metal oven racks for 10 minutes. Then, reduce the oven heat to as low as possible, prop open the oven door with a wooden or oven-safe spoon, and let the jerky dry for up to 8 hours.

<u>Weekly Schedule:</u>

The best and most optimized way to eat on a carnivorous diet is to incorporate some sort of overnight intermittent fast in order to maximize your ketosis and weight loss. Intermittent fasting might sound scary, but it's actually incredibly effective, and you won't have to stop eating at all. Most carnivorous eaters also practice intermittent fasting in order to speed up their ketosis, and they do so on a popular ratio of 16:8. These numbers indicate that you should fast for 16 hours, including your overnight fast, plus a few hours through the morning. During an 8-hour period in between noon and 8:00 p.m., you can eat whatever you want. Most carnivore diets can pack three full meals into eat hours, and leave you empty enough to enjoy a deep night's sleep. You'll be eating your first week of meals on a 16:8 schedule which, when paired with the proper preparation techniques, will ensure a steady and effective weight loss that's more significant than your carnivorous peers. When it comes to snacking, you shouldn't feel bad about failing to eat your snacks if you aren't hungry in the first place. Listen to your body, and if you aren't hungry, stick your extra snacks in the fridge or freezer to last until the following week.

MONDAY

Breakfast: 1:00   – Grilled Flank Steak

Lunch: 2:00 p.m.   – Salmon Fillets

Dinner: 6:00 p.m.   – Pork Tenderloin

Snack: – Hard-boiled Eggs.

Aim to snack either between 2:00 p.m. and 6:00 p.m. or 6:00 p.m. and 8:00 p.m. Early morning gym-goers should stick to snacking between dinner and lunch, which late night gym-goers should snack after dinner.

TUESDAY

Breakfast: 12 noon – Classic Bacon & Egg Breakfast

Lunch: 2:00 p.m.   – Bison Meatballs

Dinner: 6:00 p.m.   – Lamb Chops

Snack: – Beef Jerky

WEDNESDAY

Breakfast: 12:00   – Grilled Flank Steak

Lunch: 2:00 p.m.   – Salmon Fillets

Dinner: 6:00 p.m.   – Pork Tenderloin

Snack: – Hard-boiled Eggs

THURSDAY

Breakfast: 12:00   – Classic Bacon & Egg
Breakfast

Lunch: 2:00 p.m.   – Bison Meatballs

Dinner: 6:00 p.m.   – Lamb Chops

Snack: – Beef Jerky

FRIDAY

Breakfast: 12:00   – Grilled Flank Steak

Lunch: 2:00 p.m.   – Salmon Fillets

Dinner: 6:00 p.m.   – Pork Tenderloin

Snack: – Hard-boiled Eggs

SATURDAY

Breakfast: 12:00   – Classic Bacon & Egg
Breakfast

Lunch: 2:00 p.m.   – Charcuterie Board Social
Lunch

Dinner: 6:00 p.m   – Weekend dinner out

Snack: – Beef Jerky

SUNDAY

Breakfast: 12:00   – Smoked Salmon & sharp white cheddar roll-ups

Lunch: 2:00 p.m.   – Leftover Lamb chops

Dinner: 6:00 p.m.   – Protein shake plus pre-week meal prep leftovers and hard-boiled eggs.

FINAL NOTES

I would like to take the opportunity to thank you for reading the carnivore diet. I truly hope that you have found the information within this book useful and that it will serve you well in your journey to fulfilling your nutrition and fitness ambitions and that this is the turning point in you releasing your inner carnivore.

As I'm sure you're aware, the success of any book or author is highly dependent on its message reaching its audience, that's why I would like to ask you to review this book from the place where you purchased it, and if you know someone that you believe would benefit from this book, then please consider giving this as a gift.

I would like to thank you again for taking the time to read this book, and I truly wish you all the best in your new journey.

Robert F. Durant, 2019

We hope that you have enjoyed this book.

Original text by Robert F. Durant, 2019.

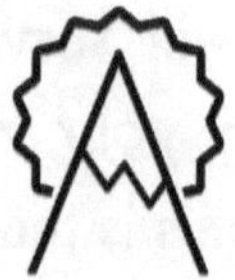

ZENITH PUBLISHING